CHOOSING OR LOSING HEALTH?

David J. Hunter

Professor of Health Policy and Management,
University of Durham

The Inaugural Haygarth Public Health Lecture,
delivered at the Crewe Hall Hotel, Crewe,
on 6 October 2005

Chester Academic Press

First published 2006
by Chester Academic Press
University of Chester
Parkgate Road
Chester CH1 4BJ

Printed and bound in the UK by the
Learning Resources Print Unit
University of Chester

Cover designed by the
Learning Resources Graphics Team
University of Chester

The Haygarth Lecture © David J. Hunter, 2006
Foreword © John Ashton, 2006

All Rights Reserved
No part of this publication may be reproduced, stored in a retrieval system or transmitted in any form or by any means without the prior permission of the copyright owner, other than as permitted by current UK legislation or under the terms of a recognised copyright licensing scheme

A catalogue record for this publication is available from the British Library

ISBNs: 1-905929-02-1 (10 digit); 978-1-905929-02-3 (13 digit)

Foreword

Professor John Ashton, CBE

Ladies and Gentlemen, I am delighted to welcome you to the inaugural Haygarth Public Health Lecture, which has been established to celebrate the long tradition of public health action in Cheshire. The lecture is named in honour of the 18th century physician John Haygarth, who practised medicine at Chester Infirmary and has been described as "Clinical Investigator and Apostle of Sanitation". The lecture is one of a series of Public Health Lectures which have been developed across the North West of England.

This inaugural lecture has a special significance in that we are also celebrating the new status of the University of Chester.

John Haygarth was born in Yorkshire in 1740. He practised as a physician in Chester and was physician to the Chester Infirmary from 1767 to 1798. It was in Chester that Haygarth first conceived and carried out his plan of treating fever patients in separate wards or hospitals.

In 1774, a census of Chester was carried out under his direction, in which he propounded seven questions about the onset and spread of two fevers which had prevailed that year.

In a paper entitled "Observations on the Population and Diseases of Chester in 1774", printed in the *Philosophical Transactions* for 1778, Haygarth suggested the removal of poor persons seized with fever to separate fever wards, spacious and airy.

In subsequent years, he obtained much accurate information about the spread of smallpox. In 1784, he published *An inquiry how to prevent the small-pox* and in

1793, *A sketch of a plan to exterminate the casual small-pox from Great Britain, and to introduce general inoculation*. These books were superseded in a few years by Jenner's discovery of vaccination.

In 1783, Haygarth's plan of separate fever wards was adopted during an epidemic in Chester. The progress of the epidemic was thus checked and he was instrumental in introducing his system into other towns.

He was one of the first to distinguish the different kinds of fevers by their periods of incubation.

It was his analysis of the diseases of Chester that led Haygarth to propose the formation in Chester of "The Smallpox Society", which was duly set up in 1778. He proposed that the technique of inoculation against the smallpox should be promoted on a large scale, and that it should also be accompanied by "Rules for Prevention".

He stressed that patients should be isolated, that no one who had not had the disease should enter the house of any victim, that no patient should be allowed out after the pocks had appeared, that the utmost attention to cleanliness was absolutely essential, and that everything to do with the patient's illness must be meticulously washed. The results were so striking that Leeds and Liverpool followed Haygarth's example.

It was at this time that Haygarth persuaded his colleagues to set up separate fever wards in the Chester Infirmary. The fever wards were an immediate success. The transmission of fevers within the hospital was effectively arrested, and at the same time fever did not spread elsewhere in the hospital. The Chester experience was the touchstone that led to the formation of fever hospitals in Manchester, Liverpool and later London.

Haygarth retired from Chester in 1798 and moved to Bath, where he lived until his death in 1827. He was 87 years old.

It is a particular pleasure for me to introduce this first Public Health Lecture associated with the new University of Chester since, for many years when I was teaching at the Liverpool Medical School, I was responsible for overseeing the quality of the Health Degrees at the then Chester College. It has been a source of satisfaction to see that work come of age and to be able to place Cheshire, together with the Universities at Chester and Keele, on a par with other parts of our emerging Regional Public Health system. I am sure that we are going to see great work in the future, which will build on the tradition that Haygarth established in the 18th century.

Turning now to a modern day public health champion, it is my enormous pleasure to welcome Professor David Hunter as our inaugural Haygarth Lecturer. David has been Professor of Health Policy and Management at the University of Durham since 2000. From 1989 to 1999, he was Professor of Health Policy and Management at the University of Leeds, and was Director of the Nuffield Institute for Health at Leeds for most of this time.

In April 2004, David took over as Chair of the UK Public Health Association. He was previously Chair of its Conferences Committee.

David is an Honorary Member of the Faculty of Public Health and a Fellow of the Royal College of Physicians of Edinburgh, and has published widely on health policy and management topics. His latest book, *Public Health Policy*, was published by Polity Press in 2003.

The Haygarth Lecture

Professor David J. Hunter

I am both flattered and privileged to have been invited to give the inaugural Haygarth Public Health Lecture for Cheshire this evening. It is an indication of how far public health has been "modernized" that a non-clinician can give such a lecture.

There is little in common between John Haygarth's career and my own, except that we both studied at Edinburgh University (he, medicine and I, political science) and share a concern with health inequalities. And it is Haygarth's concern with the health of the poor in Chester, and later in London, especially the high mortality rate from fever, that is the connecting thread between his life's work and the theme of my lecture. A second connection can be found in the link between medicine and politics. In the words of Rudolf Virchow, the famous Prussian pathologist turned anthropologist: "Medicine is a social science and politics nothing but medicine on a grand scale".

Public health is at a crossroads – yet again! For as long as I can remember – certainly since the first National Health Service [NHS] reorganization in 1974, when public health was taken away from local government – public health has been at a crossroads. But the crossroads it now finds itself at will arguably prove to be the most significant and treacherous to navigate.

The structure of my talk is in three parts:

- Public Health at a Crossroads;
- Public Health Policy: Trends and Developments;
- Public Health: Renaissance or False Dawn?

Public Health at a Crossroads

Some 15 years ago, Julio Frenk, now Minister for Health in Mexico, but then a Professor of Public Health, contributed to a book called *The Crisis in Public Health* (1992), published by the Pan American Health Organization, the Pan American Sanitary Bureau and the World Health Organization. Writing on the new public health, he argued:

> Public health has historically been one of the vital forces leading to ... collective action for health and well-being.
>
> The widespread impression exists today that this leading role has been weakening and that public health is experiencing a severe identity crisis, as well as a crisis of organization and accomplishment. (Frenk, 1992, p. 68)

My thesis is that the severe identity crisis being experienced by public health is a consequence of a shift in public policy from a concern with the collective to the individual, and from public service to markets as a means of organizing and delivering health and care (Fotaki & Boyd, 2005; Hunter 2005a, 2005b). These public policy developments have profound implications for public health and risk recreating the conditions back in the late 1700s that John Haygarth had to contend with and fought.

Society is changing and rapidly. The following health and societal trends are evident and all have a direct bearing on the public health function and how it might best be discharged:

- From a welfare to a market state;
- From central leadership to local autonomy;

- From paternalism to consumerism;
- The changing role and scope of the public realm;
- A low trust in science and experts.

What I have called the "marketization" of public health has a number of defining features:

- The language of choice;
- The reliance on the individual and the transfer of risk;
- The relationship between state and citizen, which is thinner, more transactional and contingent;
- Consumerism is preferred to collectivism;
- Work and relationships are transient;
- Short-termism prevails in work and politics;
- Public-private partnerships in the delivery of policies.

I shall return to these issues later. But I want to pause here because, while all these forces are at work at the same time, we are also being assured that public health's time has finally come, occupying a place at the top of the policy agenda. Often, this comment is made in the context of having sorted the NHS out, thereby providing the opportunity to focus upstream. But does anyone really believe that this is the case, especially in the light of the restructuring underway in the NHS – the third major reform under the Government since 1997 – and the financial deficits that are mounting?

Public Health Policy: Trends and Developments

The health challenges of the 21st century are principally public health challenges, in respect of chronic diseases which are preventable, and pandemics, like avian bird flu, which have yet fully to test our systems (although there is great concern that these will be overwhelmed and we will be unable to cope if a truly potent pandemic occurs – see, for instance, Laurie Garrett's paper in the July/August 2005 issue of *Foreign Affairs*). In October 2005, *The Lancet* carried a series of articles on global chronic disease, under the heading, "The Neglected Epidemic". In 2005 alone, 35 million people will die from heart disease, stroke, cancer and other chronic diseases. Most of them will be in low and middle-income countries (Strong, Mathers, Leeder, & Beaglehole, 2005).

We also know that health inequalities between social groups are widening in all countries, including the UK, and that public health has much to contribute to their resolution, as well as other public policies designed to minimize the wealth gap (Mackenbach, 2005). Indeed, it is argued that, if we focused on the wealth gap rather than the health gap, then health would largely take care of itself.

Back in 1997, with the arrival of a new government and one refreshingly predisposed to talk about health and inequalities in health, there was a mood of optimism and hope. Not only was the first ever public health minister appointed in England, but a new health strategy was crafted. When *Saving Lives: Our Healthier Nation* finally appeared in 1999, it was a little disappointing, but it did acknowledge the importance of tackling the social determinants of health and government's central role in this endeavour. Sadly, the impetus behind public health seemed to dissipate, as the NHS Plan in 2000 assumed centre stage and the Government became preoccupied with downstream issues affecting the acute care sector. Waiting lists, beds and access dominated the policy agenda.

Rediscovery of Public Health

It was not until Derek Wanless was asked by the Treasury in 2001 to consider the likely challenges that might befall the NHS over a 20-year period up to 2022 that public health began to reassert itself and be rediscovered (Wanless, 2002). Indeed, the Government rushed to sign up to the "fully engaged" scenario, the most ambitious of the three scenarios put forward by Wanless. And it is not hard to figure out why. Underlying this scenario, alongside productivity gains in the NHS, was the assumption that the public would be fully engaged with their health and take greater responsibility for it. Were this nirvana to be achieved, the prize for the Treasury would be a £30 million saving on NHS expenditure per year, although a large proportion of such savings would be achieved through productivity gains in health care.

Needless to say, the Chancellor wanted to know how successful we were being in implementing the fully engaged scenario and invited Wanless back to take a look and report on progress. In his second report, specifically on public health, Wanless went further in his critique of policy failure (Wanless, 2004). His report triggered the 2004 English public health White Paper, *Choosing Health*, and all that flows from it. So what did he say? His critique can be distilled into the following key points:

- The NHS remains a "sickness" rather than a "health" service;
- The failure over 30 years to bring about change;
- The key challenge is delivery and implementation;
- The public health workforce is "not fit for purpose";
- The weak capacity of Primary Care Trusts to deliver;

- The poor state of the evidence base and underinvestment in Research & Development;
- The health literacy of the population is poor.

Perhaps Wanless's most pointed criticism was reserved for what he saw as consistent failure on the part of successive governments over 30 years to implement the many worthy policy statements that had been produced. The problem was not lack of policy, but a failure to implement it. This excerpt admirably sums up his argument:

> Numerous policy statements and initiatives in the field of public health have not resulted in a rebalancing of policy away from health care (a "national sickness service") to health (a "national health service"). This will not happen until there is a realignment of incentives in the system to focus on reducing the burden of disease and tackling the key lifestyle and environmental risks. (Wanless, 2004, p. 23)

In its White Paper, the Government proclaims that it means business this time and that action will follow. But what sort of action? It seems that, between 1999 and 2004, the role of government itself in protecting the population's health underwent something of a quiet revolution. This is what health ministers were saying in 1999, in their new health strategy, which "… will require action by Government, by local organizations and by individuals. Some of the factors which harm people's health are beyond the control of any single individual" (Secretary of State for Health, 1999, Preface). The foreword to the consultation paper, *Our Healthier Nation*, went further in stressing the role of government: "Now we want to see far more attention and Government action concentrated on the things which damage people's health" (Secretary of State for Health, 1998, p. 2).

Contrast these words with what the Prime Minister said in 2004: "We are clear that Government cannot ... pretend it can 'make' the population healthy. But it can - and should – support people in making better choices for their health ..." (Secretary of State for Health, 2004, p. 3).

It is perhaps unfair to read too much into selected quotations and the Government's new public health strategy does contain some positive features, including:

- A focus on health promotion;
- A key role for the NHS in promoting health;
- Planned Local Area Agreements;
- Action on physical activity, obesity, smoking and food standards;
- Better use of the workforce; e.g. in pharmacy and dentistry;
- A focus on evidence and information;
- A strengthening of workforce capacity and capability.

We should not lose sight of these. However, the weaknesses of the approach are considerable, arguably more problematic, and need to be addressed because, unless they are, the positive aspects may never emerge or may simply fall short of the response required. The key weaknesses in my view are these:

- The absence of sound leadership from central government;
- No mention of a Minister for Public Health;
- Health inequalities receive little mention;

- Underlying health determinants are ignored;
- Local government is marginalized;
- There is a fixation on individual choice rather than healthy public policy;
- Is the strategy in fact about public health at all?

This last point – is the White Paper about public health at all? – goes to the nub of the issue and to the changes in ideology that appear to have gripped the Government since about 2002. But, before elaborating on these, it is important to emphasize just how unequal British society still is, despite the Government's efforts since 1997. For example, the Institute for Public Policy Research [IPPR], in a recent audit of injustice in the UK, concluded that Britain is far from being a just society. In particular: "Levels of child poverty continue to surpass those of many of our more successful European partners and inequalities in income, wealth and well-being remain stubbornly high" (Paxton & Dixon, 2004, p. 5). Social mobility appears to have declined in the UK, although it has increased in other European countries, including France, the Netherlands and Sweden. A social class gap remains a divisive feature in the UK. Although an aggregate improvement in educational attainment has been achieved, the higher level of entry into higher education has benefited the well-off more than the poor. Regional inequalities remain high. In the South East, 17% of people are in the poorest 20% of the population, compared with 26% of people in the North East. The position is worse if Scotland is included: there, eight out of 10 local authorities with the lowest male life expectancy are located.

We also have more recent confirmation of these trends from the Government itself, in the Marmot Report, slipped out in mid-August (Department of Health, 2005). Against the backdrop of these societal developments and trends, the principles underlying *Choosing Health* seem rather feeble and unambitious, and fall far short of the response required:

- Informed choice;
- Personalization;
- Working together.

Instead, a more challenging set of principles might be those which underpin the UK Public Health Association's mission:

- Combating health inequalities;
- Promoting sustainable development;
- Challenging anti-health forces.

To tackle the public health problems we face, there surely needs to be an inter-sectoral approach at all levels of government, from the individual to the global. For all its rhetoric, it is not evident that the Government is truly committed to such a joined-up vertical and horizontal approach.

The central flaw in the White Paper is that it puts the focus firmly on the individual. Why? The reasons are complex and multi-faceted. In an attempt to offer an explanation, or at least a partial one, let me return to the start of the lecture, when I referred to the importance of the crossroads at which public health once again finds itself. I described a number of trends that appear to be in the ascendant and perhaps define the Government's overall stance when it comes to public sector reform.

These trends place a heavy reliance on markets and competition in the execution of public policy. But the market state which is gripping governments and public policy around the world offers no panacea and is riven with its own paradoxes. Philip Bobbitt, in his epic book *The Shield of Achilles* (2002, p. 234), singles out three of them for special mention:

- *"It will require more centralized authority for government* [italics added], but all governments will be weaker", as they devolve, contract out or withdraw altogether from activities;
- *"There will be more public participation in government* [italics added], but it will count for less", with the role of citizen as activist diminishing and the role as spectator increasing;
- *"The welfare state will have greatly retrenched* [italics added], but infrastructure security, epidemiological surveillance and environmental protection" will be promoted by government as never before.

I would venture to suggest that each of these paradoxes is already in evidence to some degree.

The risks of the marketization of public policy are considerable in respect of health and health care systems. They include the following:

- The fragmentation of health care;
- The loss of integration and joined-up policy;
- Chronic disease and public health demand a "whole systems" response;
- Public governance and private markets – governments lack the capacity to manage relationships;
- The high cost of regulation – the danger of "mission creep";
- Cost inflation, as new private monopolies emerge;

- There can be no turning back once the genie is out of the bottle.

Underlying these developments, which appear to be ideologically inspired rather than the result of looking at the evidence, is an assault on the public realm. David Marquand, who has written extensively on the hollowing out of the state and the loss of the public realm, articulates two conceptions of modernity (Marquand, 2005, p. 335):

> One is the managerial, economistic, deterministic and top-down conception implicit in the Washington Consensus, cherished by global businesses, increasingly espoused by public sector managers who ought to know better, and propagated by most of the media and all three mainstream political parties .... The other is a humanistic, decentralist, "green", and pluralistic conception, which commands increasing support in civil society, particularly among the young, but is almost squeezed out of formal politics.

It is clearly the first conception which dominates public discourse.

Recalling the quotation from Julio Frenk with which I opened this lecture, I would argue that the identity crisis being experienced by public health has much to do with the loss of confidence in the public realm. It has left those practising public health somewhat adrift. Hitherto, no clear or convincing case has been put in favour of what the public realm might, or should, look like in future. This vacuum presents public health with a serious dilemma, since by definition its work is carried out in the public sphere and lies outside a market framework.

I believe that the increasing marketization of public policy (and one need look no further than the NHS for evidence of this) cannot simply be ignored as a passing whim or fad. It goes to the heart of the neo-liberal consensus emerging across many countries in the West and I have described its key elements. In short, health is to be defined and marketed in terms of personal fitness, body imagery and individual achievement. For confirmation of these trends, one need look no further than the burgeoning craze for cosmetic surgery in the UK.

Public Health: Renaissance or False Dawn?

I do not have a simple or unequivocal answer to this question. The optimist in me would veer to the renaissance view, but the realist verging on pessimist in me fears another false dawn, of which we have witnessed so many in public health. The challenge the public health community faces is huge if another false dawn is to be avoided. It includes the following features:

- An inverse care law is still alive;
- An inverse preventive care law is alive;
- There is a need for sustained political will and commitment;
- The stewardship role of government versus the role of the individual;
- Many (perhaps most) of the influences on health lie outside the policy domain of health departments;
- The need for an outcomes-led approach to health;
- A culture shift is required in the NHS.

Many risks are present, especially when the public health lead remains harnessed to the fate of the NHS. Among them are the following:

- The pull of the acute sector remains strong;
- Public health is reduced to health education and promotion;
- Resources for public health do not materialize;
- The increasing medicalization of public health problems.

Perhaps the current "redisorganization" of the NHS will offer the opportunity to rethink where public health should be located. For many, a return to local government looks attractive. However, the issue should not be seen in structural or organizational terms, but rather in terms of where a public health mindset can most profitably take root.

The key to good public health lies in sustainable development. The two agendas need to be linked in an attempt to rediscover the public realm and to make collective action fashionable again. There needs to be a coherent public health system, of which the NHS would form a part – a point John Ashton made in his Milroy Lecture in 2000 (Ashton, 2004). In the face of some resistance, I have no doubt, this will mean removing lead responsibility for the public's health from the silo of the NHS.

Finally, effective leadership is required at a government level to challenge anti-health forces. Government needs to play industry at its own game and be smarter. Legislation should be introduced to control advertising to children, the smoking ban should apply to all workplaces, and education in schools should include positive health approaches.

So, having scoped the problem and dilemmas facing public health, I leave you to come up with your own answer to the question: "Are we witnessing a public health renaissance or another false dawn?" Maybe the White

Paper's closing words will help you: "This is the beginning of a journey to build health into Government policy and ensure that health is everybody's business" (Secretary of State for Health, 2004, p. 181).

Or maybe not! In fact, it seems that health is some people's business more than others, as it indicates a retreat from enlightened government action that resulted in, for example, seat belt legislation, and has enabled many countries, including the rest of the UK, before England finally and somewhat reluctantly fell into line, to legislate for smoke-free public places. Simply offering people information and education to change lifestyles, as well as the services of a health trainer (whatever and whoever they may be), will not result in healthier eating habits or the uptake of physical exercise regimes. There are societal and infrastructural issues that need to be addressed too, and only government at local, regional and national levels can do this.

Conclusion

Let me conclude. The central paradox for public policy is that, at precisely the time public health has risen up the policy agenda, it has become subjected to the neo-liberal embrace that is narrowing the focus of public health and placing responsibility for it increasingly at the personal level. Yet, at the same time, the determinants of health and the most powerful means for health improvement are increasingly located at local, regional, national and global levels.

Above all, the public health community's voice needs to be heard as an advocate for sustained political will and for government's stewardship role to be championed. This means acknowledging, too, the importance of the public realm. There are limits to markets and to viewing individuals as consumers, exercising unfettered choice. It is time those concerned about the public's health acknowledged these and acted accordingly. Public health practitioners, as one commentator observed, are good at measuring risk behaviour and counting the dead; but much more is needed to improve health.

In a recent editorial published in the *British Medical Journal*, Ilona Kickbusch (2005, July 30, p. 246) wrote: "… health is deeply political. We need to tackle the political determinants of health. National public health associations and medical associations should be at the forefront of explaining and exploring the interface of national and global public health agendas …". She urged them to: "… commit to this unique historical opportunity, which is on a par to the big steps undertaken in the 19th century golden age of public health".

I think John Haygarth would have approved and gone along with this call to action. We must, too.

Thank you!

References

Ashton, J. (2004). *State medicine and public hygiene: Implication of the new public health: Milroy Lecture 2000.* Liverpool: Centre for Public Health.

Bobbitt, P. (2002). *The shield of Achilles: War, peace and the course of history.* London: Allen Lane.

Department of Health. (2005). *Tackling health inequalities: Status report on the Programme for Action.* London: Author.

Fotaki, K., & Boyd, A. (2005). From plan to market: A comparison of health and old age care policies in the UK and Sweden. *Public Money and Management, 25* (4), 237-243.

Frenk, J. (1992). The new public health. In *The crisis of public health: Reflections for the debate* (pp. 68-85). Washington, DC: Pan American Health Organization, Pan American Sanitary Bureau, Regional Office of the World Health Organization.

Garrett, L. (1995, July/August). The next pandemic? [Electronic version]. *Foreign Affairs,* 1-8.

Hunter, D. J. (2005a). Choosing or losing health? *Journal of Epidemiology and Community Health, 59* (12), 1010-1012.

Hunter, D. J. (2005b). The fall and rise of the NHS. *PMPA Review, 31,* 12-13.

Kickbusch, I. (2005, July 30). Tackling the political determinants of global health. *British Medical Journal, 331,* 246-7.

Mackenbach, J. (2005). *Health inequalities: Europe in profile.* London: Central Office of Information, for the UK Presidency of the EU.

Marquand, D. (2005). Monarchy, state and dystopia. *The Political Quarterly, 76* (3), 333-336.

Paxton, W., & Dixon, M. (2004). *The state of the nation: an audit of injustice in the UK.* London: Institute for Public Policy Research.

Secretary of State for Health. (1998). *Our healthier nation: A contract for health* (Cm 3852). London: The Stationery Office.

Secretary of State for Health. (1999). *Saving lives: Our healthier nation* (Cm 4386). London: The Stationery Office.

Secretary of State for Health. (2004). *Choosing health: Making healthy choices easier* (Cm 6374). London: The Stationery Office.

Strong, K., Mathers, C., Leeder, S., & Beaglehole, R. (2005, October 29). Preventing chronic diseases: how many lives can we save? *The Lancet, 366,* 1578-1582.

Wanless, D. (2002). *Securing our future health: Taking a long-term view: Final report.* London: HM Treasury.

Wanless, D. (2004). *Securing good health for the whole population: Final report.* London: The Stationery Office.